Here's The Deal

Healthy Weight Loss
and
Fat Burning Over 40

Megan C. Scott

Disclaimer:

This book is not intended as a substitute for the medical advice of physicians. The information, stories and articles contained in this book are the opinion of the individual author based on her personal observations and years of experience. Neither the author nor the publisher assume any liability whatsoever for the use of or inability to use any or all information contained in this book.

Free Bonus Gift

Before you read any further, be sure to snag your delicious *free DEAL recipes PDF* featuring some of the most highly rated recipes from the original DEAL book plus a few as-yet unpublished gems!

I certainly don't want you to miss out on Homemade Chocolate Bar Bliss, Peachy Dream Smoothie, or SweetHeat Veggie Asian Stir Fry along with many more!

Click below to snag your free recipes and also get notifications of upcoming new cookbook releases, healthy recipes, tips and encouragement for your journey!

https://healthyweightlossandfatburning.com/BonusRecipesGift

TABLE OF CONTENTS

Introduction

Hi - I'm Megan, and I am over 40. And I'm so glad you are here!

I want you to know that I truly understand the struggle to lose weight - or keep it off - and like you, I am keenly aware of those late night cravings and yearnings for just a few more bites of something delicious to drown out some of the chaos of the day. We deserve it, right? Well, we also deserve to feel and look our best and love life at the same time! Enjoying food does not mean we can't have a healthy body!

So now I invite you to join me as we take an honest look at healthy weight loss that works. You can count on me to show you the real DEAL and encourage you along the way as well. We're in this together, and I sense victory just around the corner for both of us!

Your Body Real Estate: A Word Picture

*Y*our body is your personal real estate. It can be as clean or as cluttered as you allow it to be. Think with me for a moment about planning to sell your current home.

Would you show your home with piles of clutter in every room? What do you think that would do to the value of your home?

I lived in a previous house that needed to be appraised to calculate the market value. There wasn't a lot of time before the appraiser was coming, so cleanup was quick and not "deep" - not Spring cleaning, by any stretch! You might say it was straightened up and cleaned with a "lick and a promise". Did that make any difference in the end result?

Well, let me say that I was very disappointed in the appraiser's estimate of the home's value. I thought the appraiser would primarily look at the structure itself, the rooms and storage, and the condition of the home inside and out. But he didn't seem to see it the way I did.

Rather than giving up, I decided to have it reappraised and do some really deep cleaning on that home! I asked my sister to come and help (she is an organizing guru!) and we spent a large number of hours making that place sparkle! We didn't have time to make decision after decision about what to do with clutter in the basement (some of which didn't even belong to me!), so my sister got a few dozen large black trash bags and started throwing stuff into them. All of the bags were tossed neatly one upon the other in one small part of the basement. The rest was cleaned up very neatly (most of the basement was unfinished).

The appraiser returned a few weeks later. What happened?

A shining, spotless home made a HUGE first impression, and the entire feeling of the place was changed. Everything neat and in it's place; dust gone, shiny floors and de-cluttering made an almost unbelievable difference. If you can fathom this, the house was re-appraised at about $20,000 higher than it was previously!! Amazing!

So what about your body real estate? Are you improving it? Or are you anesthetized to it, like the piles of clutter you rarely notice in your closet or garage? The results of "letting things go" is clutter and disarray. And excess fat is really just body clutter!

I've read a book recently called The Compound Effect. The entire gist of the book is that BIG changes can take place with small incremental changes maintained over time. The same is true for your body! And did you know that there is a relationship between axing household or office clutter and weight loss? Once your surroundings become clean and uncluttered, you'll be amazed at how you'll begin to think differently about other areas of your life as well.

If you think about it, clutter is "stuff" that's either useless or out of place. It detracts from the feeling of orderliness and productivity of any particular room. It's not a far stretch to see our bodies in similar fashion. "Extra" fat, rolls, or skin that's "out of place" tends to detract from the beauty of the person that is you! You're still that amazing person inside, but releasing that leaner "you" can add an incredible amount of productivity to your day as well as a calm to your life. Whether with house clutter or body clutter, when we finally get down to business to create a healthier space, it's amazing how focused we can become.

When you decide to move from your home, all of a sudden you become very AWARE of how your home looks - inside and outside, room by room. It is that AWARENESS that motivates you to "see your house as an outsider would" and make it as attractive as you can.

The first key to healthy weight and fat loss (and "getting into shape" as we call it) is to become AWARE of how you really look (measurements, pictures) and how you really FEEL, and then tracking what you eat and how you feel subsequently. You need to know what really IS before you're ready to determine what WILL BE in the future. No rose colored glasses allowed!

DEALING With What Is

Awareness

*Y*es, the first real step to change is AWARENESS - just like it is when you are cleaning your home for company, or deep cleaning it and repainting, repairing, etc. for showing your home in hopes that you will find a buyer quickly.

Where the comparison ends is that when it comes to "body real estate", you will not be recreating your body primarily for others - although they may be somewhat of a factor (you want to live to see your children grow up, you want to have energy to take care of your family, etc.).

But your primary "why" needs to come from deep within. What will motivate YOU to stick with your plan? I want you to imagine yourself 6 months - 1 year from now. How will you be feeling in your new, trimmer and leaner body? How will your life have improved for the better because you decided to DEAL with the problem instead of allowing "body clutter" to take over your life and personal space?

Write it Down

Now I want you to **write this down.** And I want you to write it - not just as an "I want to" statement, but to write down your results as if you have already achieved them. Project yourself 6 months into the future. What will you look and feel like then?

This is a powerful exercise that engages your emotions, will and imagination!

Here's my example:

I got serious about my body clutter this year and I have the results to prove it! I am amazed when I look in the mirror, and I love what I see. I have lost 20 pounds, and (believe it or not) 50 inches!! I am exercising 3-4 times a week - doing what I love - and I feel so good there's no stopping me now! I have learned to cook healthier meals, I am learning to dehydrate living foods, and I'm adding more fresh fruits and vegetables to my diet. I feel so awesome, that it's hard to imagine how I existed before with so much lethargy, bloat and exhaustion. I have the energy to play with my grandkids, I like to go out with my friends in the evenings occasionally, and my living space is transformed as well! I feel so much better, I look so much better, and my actions show that I am now full of life, instead of just "full of food". I love my life!

See how powerful this is? Please do not skip this part - take a few minutes RIGHT NOW to write down what you want your life to be like in 6 months - don't let the "what ifs" stand in your way, either (I know what you're thinking!).

If, for example, your initial goals are similar to mine - and you hit the 6-month mark and have lost 15 pounds and 20 inches, that is not failing - it's a TREMENDOUS success! But it's vital to state what you want in "right now" words, and paint that future you want to create. Your body and mind will begin to line up with what you confess to be true!

As a powerful Scripture verse states:

"As a man (woman) thinks in his heart, so is he (she)."

It works if you work it - consistently!

You might even want to post your "future you" word picture in a prominent place, or put it in a special book where you can read it every day. Keep the vision in front of you! It will motivate and inspire you to stick with it when the going gets tough.

Now of course, just willpower, or "wishful thinking" won't get you very far. So in the rest of this book I'm going to outline a simple plan that can keep you on track to reach your "new body" goals. You can do this!

Here's the DEAL

The Real Deal

DEAL -
D – Detox (detoxification)
E - Exercise
A - Action Tracking
L - Low Carb

$\mathcal{F}$eeling bloated and fat after the Holiday Celebrations? Ate too much wedding cake at that reception? Need to clean out all the junk food before you start your 32nd diet of the last 10 years?

Let's face it - We Boomers particularly tend to be very responsible people - we don't want to "waste" anything - particularly food. This is probably due to the fact that our parents or grandparents lived during the great Depression in the 1930s, and were terrified to run out of anything - nothing can be wasted!

Excuses, Excuses

So our ultra-responsibility kicks in, and we tell ourselves things like:

"Mom said to finish everything on my plate because children are starving every day in Africa." (Maybe not telling ourselves ALOUD, but the thought stream is there, nonetheless!)

"Just a few more cookies to go, and this batch will be history and I can go back on my diet (eating plan, healthy lifestyle, etc.).

"Well, I lost 5 pounds in the months preceding Christmas, and I only gained 5 during the season, so at least I'm not 10 pounds heavier!!" (Let's call it even)

But even "even" makes us feel sluggish, tired, overweight, and generally "not good" about ourselves.

You see, the reason all of the "waste" talk doesn't help is simply this;

If we are convinced the food shouldn't go to waste - and we eat it - it still goes to WAIST!!! Ours, in particular!

So what is the answer?

I listened to a webinar (a seminar on the Internet) just yesterday on goal setting for the upcoming year, and the organizer said something very compelling. Even if we haven't STARTED our new plan yet, just committing to do something - in writing - can make us feel better. Because now we have a PLAN and a goal and we know we are going to take action towards it. So, as I lay awake in the middle of the night last evening, I came up with a plan. You can track with me and create your own plan from this simple model. We all know that consistency is the key to breakthrough in any area of life, right? Even small actions, taken consistently over time will yield good - and even great results over an extended period of time.

So here's the DEAL:

Probably a vast majority of the population - Baby Boomers in particular - are looking for weight loss answers when the

New Year is coming (or summer, or the change of seasons, or a family or high school reunion, or.... you get the picture).

So we're going to work WITH that natural tendency. But you're going to have the opportunity to CUSTOMIZE the program to YOU and your needs.

Why Most "One Size Fits All" Programs Are Doomed To Fail

Here's the scoop - most of us tend to be rather undisciplined when it comes to eating and exercise. So it naturally seems easier to buy a program (think of that one advertised on TV where you have meals and snacks delivered to your door for your weight loss without worry!) The thing is, this kind of pre-packaged program can take a HUGE bite out of your wallet. And what happens when you can no longer afford a few hundred a month to keep the butler service arriving at your front door on cue? Will you still be losing weight and just as motivated?

I think I can glimpse a doubtful look in your eye! I know myself - if somebody is doing all the work FOR me and then I can no longer afford it, am I likely to take that all on myself? Well, Nooooooooooo.So I have a better solution for us Baby Boomers and Generation X folks who are weary of our non-svelte figures and our lack of time to dedicate hours a day or hundreds of dollars a month for this potion, or that meal plan, or the latest Yoga/Tai-Chi/Power Lifting/$99 Karate Course those convincing sales page writers have so graciously written for our tired, overworked, and desperate brains (which, by the way, are attached to those not - so - svelte bodies we're sporting around). I know - long sentence - but can you relate to that?

Discover your WHY

The truth is, your reasons to lose and get into shape must be stronger than your poor habits of eating whatever and whenever you feel like it. Reread the previous section on why you want to get into shape. What did you write down?

I've decided on a goal for myself - I have a business conference in 3 weeks, and I want to lose 10 pounds (including the 5 I gained back that I had worked so hard to lose).

I'm breaking it down to the smallest picture I can.

10 pounds in 3 weeks would mean losing 8 ounces (or 1/2 pound) per day, on average, for 21 days.

And I'm not going to starve, or lose water weight or muscle. I want to lose FAT and rolls and bloat! In other words, no "pretense" weight loss where the scales show one thing but my body ends up in an unhealthy or weakened state - no thank you!

3-5 simple Steps you KNOW will work

I was inspired by a blog post last week that was talking about simply doing the things we already KNOW for a specific period of time for results - instead of buying the "latest greatest" elixir or exercise program.

Let's make a DEAL, fellow Boomers!

I know from years of experience (and study in nutrition) what kinds of things are healthy and lead to weight and fat loss, and what doesn't work. You've got some pretty good ideas yourself. So I'm going to take that blogger's advice and concentrate on 4 simple steps to get to my goals of losing this weight and fat.

My first goal is for the next 3 weeks (you can track with me) - and I will implement the ideas described in this book.

The DEAL will give you structure and a basic plan, and then you can customize it according to what you have already tried that has worked for you, and things you would like to attempt - simply track your results. My plan is to measure my results after each month, and then tweak and adapt for the following month.

Creatures of Habit and Starved for Diversion

We humans are an interesting lot. On the one hand, we are definitely creatures of habit, and we typically would rather operate on autopilot - doing what we've always done - rather than start something new and unique that requires sustained effort.

On the other hand, we are starved for diversion, so "bright shiny object" syndrome catches our attention. Most of us don't find it difficult to START something new, but the follow through is entirely another matter!

To prove my point, just think about the following:

How many diet and/or exercise programs have you started (with high motivation) that you no longer follow?

Have you retained the results of those earlier moments of effort?

Exactly.

Consistency is the key to breakthrough, and most of us have a VERY difficult time sustaining the effort required to follow someone else's exact program of how we should do this or eat that.

Because as humans, we have another inherent trait - most of us don't like someone else telling us exactly what to do. So, although we might follow along for a while, we eventually rebel because that diet developer doesn't know us, doesn't walk in our shoes, and doesn't realize how next-to-impossible these demands are! (at least over the long haul)

Let's Make a Deal

CUSTOMIZATION of the DEAL for You and You Alone

So...let's make a DEAL.

There are 4 simple things I have known for years that will contribute to weight and fat loss.

They are the DEAL:

D - Detoxification

E - Exercise

A - Action Tracking

L - Low Carbohydrate Options

Now I'm going to break these down to what I have personally tried that has been successful, or what friends and professionals have recommended to me that would improve my health.

Here are the Guidelines - You Are in Charge of the Choices!

Detox

This includes products such as detox teas, colon cleansing products (Colon Blow and Blessed Herbs are two examples), detoxing foods and herbs, and a detoxing diet.

Exercise

What do you love?

This a great place to start. My massage therapist has made specific recommendations to me to structurally support my body since I spend so much time at the computer keyboard. He told me to cut something else out of my expenses and join the YMCA and go to swimming! It is easy on the joints, and stretches the muscles in addition to being a great cardio exercise.

Do you love to bike? Recumbent biking is gaining ground as the perfect leg exercise without the strain on the midsection (postural) that regular or race biking can cause.

Perhaps it's walking or running.

Whatever it is, learn the basics of safely engaging in the exercise and then set some specific written and get to it!

Action Tracking

This one is great - and CRUCIAL!

Weigh and measure yourself before you start your program so you have a baseline to compare to. Then track what you eat - everything - and how you feel after exercise (and what you did) - and how you will tweak it as you go along

TRACK even how you *feel* after eating - or exercising - or when you are tempted to "stress eat" (like I did yesterday with spice cookies and thin mints) - what are you saying to yourself? Replace this with healthy self-talk!

A simple solution is to get a notebook and use a page per day. Write down what you eat and when, and how you feel in between (or before) you eat. I put my current weight in the top right corner so I can easily flip back through and see my progress.

L – Low Carb Food Options

Carbohydrates are great for energy, and many foods contain them. But they need to be kept in balance – and healthy carbs are what you want to implement into your eating plan. What happens if your carbs are out of balance?Too low, and your plan will be extremely hard to maintain, in addition to the real possibility of resulting health problems.Too high - you'll never meet your goals!

The Standard American diet (SAD) is high in processed carbohydrates, all of which rank highly on the glycemic index scale. This means they affect your blood sugar quickly and may even lead to diabetes. A better choice is to become familiar with low glycemic index foods - typically natural foods and whole grains - which give the blood sugar a steadier supply of nutrients.

Shoot for moderate to low carb intake on a daily basis - and have "free carb days" - but try to stick with healthy carbs. Some authors say "low carb" is 20 g a day- others say below 75 g. I personally shoot for fewer than 50, but I track how my body is responding and adjust accordingly. Again, the type of carbohydrates is all-important here!

Quick and Easy Path to a Varied 4 Step Health Routine

*C*hoose each letter of the DEAL plan - then list whatever comes to mind that would fit into this category as quickly as you can. If needed, take about 10 minutes to Google some info and add it to your list.

Then, each day, choose just ONE THING from your lists for each category.

(You can adapt this to your changing moods and energy level for a really sweet way to stay on track and still maintain your variety and your sanity!)

Here's what I chose for today for myself (to give you an idea of how easy this is):

Detox - I don't feel too hot today, so this needs to be easy. I'm going to drink a cup of herbal "Smooth Move Tea" before I go to bed this evening. (Chocolate is my favorite)

Exercise - I've been caring for my daughter post - op this week, so have had little time or energy to exercise. I've also been up through the night to give her medicine, and I lay awake for 2 hours after the first shift (which, coincidentally, was when the idea for this book was born). I feel very weary, and a bit exhausted, so the exercise today needs to be low key. I plan to do 50 stomach squeezes while laying flat in bed before I go to sleep tonight. (No lifting or crunching - Tony the massage therapist says that to gain a tummy 6- pack in due time, simply squeeze your surface stomach muscles while lying flat - it won't mess up your postural muscles that way).

Action Tracking - today, I took my initial body measurements and am also keeping a food journal. I'm noting what I'm eating - including amounts and approximate carbohydrate counts. **If you skip this important step for a number of days, it's all too easy to fall off the wagon and begin gaining back that weight - so keep on trackin'!**

Low Carb - this is top of mind for me today. I know that protein axes sugar cravings, so I just ate 3 scrambled eggs with onions, peppers, and garlic and a touch of cheese when I got hungry a few minutes ago. What I listed above is just an example. But you can see that although I am MINDFUL of what I am eating and doing and why, it is not dominating my day and my time! I'm adapting it according to my energy level and responsibilities, and yet still making forward progress. And for me, there's something INCREDIBLY ATTRACTIVE about being able to make a CHOICE - and not feeling tied down to only ONE way of eating or living that fences me in and eventually creates irritability and that rebellion mentality. Can you relate?

Try it for yourself and then track your results!
Turn the page to find out what you'll want to avoid – those pesky deal-breakers!

Deal Breakers

*I*n addition to avoiding the "Terrible Two" that have been in the news recently - Trans Fats and HFCS (High Fructose Corn Syrup), there are a few other deal breakers you will want to be aware of. Here's a short list of things you absolutely cannot expect to eat and do on a daily basis if you're serious about your weight loss goals.

List:

* Deep fried foods

* Processed foods (with items on the label you can't even pronounce!)

---- Any food that is "white" can be off limits for best results - highly processed flour, rice and sugar is difficult for the body to process, and clogs up your system {it's like running your auto on soda pop!}

* Beer

* High saturated fat foods

* Soda

* A diet heavy in breads

And be sure to avoid:

* Shortchanging your sleep

* Chronic stress in your life

* Dehydration

If you are a lover of fast food, I encourage you to Google the list of ingredients in your "favorite" foods. It just might inspire you to refrain from grabbing those unhealthy junk foods on the run!

Dealing With Deception

Artificial Sweeteners

Chemicals

Genetically modified (GMO) "foods"

Isolated vitamins (non whole food based vitamins may be made from sewage sludge!)

Stripped and ultra processed foods (white flour, white sugar, white rice)

There are multiple deception factors being perpetrated by the food industry. For instance, artificial sweeteners have been shown to actually CREATE carb cravings, according to recent research, and, if a food has been modified by either chemicals or genetic engineering, we don't know how (or if) the body is processing it effectively. I personally have stomach pains after eating Splenda, and there is some pretty frightening research out there about NutraSweet!

In addition, sometimes we deceive ourselves. We encourage all too many cheat days and meals, telling ourselves that we will lose that weight soon! We'll be feeling much slimmer, trimmer and vibrant by next year this time! There is no end to the countless little things we can tell ourselves to make us feel better in the moment.

That' s what I discovered when I reread my journal from this past year. I lost about 25 pounds.

Why in the world wasn't I happy then?

Because I lost that same 4 or 5 pounds over and over again!!

It was a fluctuation of a few pounds circling around the same main number on those scales - and I decided I was tired of pretending things would get better and just DEAL with it!

(You see, I'm taking my own prescription!)

Yes, I'm just like you. I'm a Boomer who also struggles with weight gain, sluggishness, and busy-ness that attempts to seduce me into believing that I don't really have the time to exercise.

Or to eat right. Or get into those skinny clothes again.

The difference now is, that I refuse to believe it.

The deal is, that the DEAL is working!

Here's the proof.

Report:

I went just a day over 2 weeks to record my results of following the DEAL diet (rather loosely on some days, with a family health emergency in the mix) - I lost a total of 4.8 pounds.

Not bad, eh? But it seems too slow to me!

Don't be surprised if you are anxious to lose more weight faster. This is normal. Just remember that slow and steady wins the race!

Now here's why you'll want to measure yourself before you start on the DEAL diet / lifestyle: Because you've just gotta know!

Here are the measurements to take:

(A tape measure and 3x5 card work just fine)

Bust (women)

Chest

Stomach (2" below belly button, or the largest part)
Hips
R and L thigh
R and L calf
R and L bicep

I would have been a little discouraged about losing less than 5 pounds in 2 weeks, and maybe would have given up - had I not measured previously. When I re-measured…I was both surprised - and pleased! In addition to losing nearly 5 pounds, I also lost 8 1/2 inches! 3 1/2 inches melted off of my tummy measurement alone. Now THAT provided some more "stick to it" motivation! Even though I had reached a plateau for a number of days, the inches continued to melt away. The scales can be deceiving - don't depend only on what they say! Your results may be a lot different - or they may be similar. Don't worry - just track the small changes your body is making, tweak your plan and exercise program and keep on keeping on!

As an added incentive, listen to what my wise, older sister told me. When I complained about "only" losing two pounds, she said: "That's **8 sticks of butter!**" Now Imagine losing 4 sticks of butter each time you drop a pound of fat, and I promise you'll look at your weight loss in a different light!

Just DEAL WITH IT!!

I cannot overemphasize the importance of quality decision.

$\mathcal{I}$t's true. This will be the first thing that will propel you in the direction of your new body. A quality decision backed up with solid action. The key is to not allow distractions and discouragement to affect the logic of that decision. As the famous tagline of Nike says: Just Do It!

Getting Past Discouragement

When you feel discouraged, remind yourself of the good decisions you are making. Celebrate even the smallest areas of progress. Cheer yourself on as a coach would a runner who is tiring on the track. Become your own biggest cheerleader!

Sticking With It

This one is easier than you think. Set certain actions in stone, so to speak, and don't budge from them. Make it nonnegotiable - even with yourself! Perhaps you'll give up certain foods for 30 days (or better yet, substitute them for better and amazing foods). Maybe it is 6 weeks of exercising 4 times a week or more, doing what you love. You can do this, and you don't have to feel deprived during the process!

Motivational Mojos

What will inspire you? How about walking into your closet and proclaiming that you will soon fit into that favorite pair of pants again?
Feeling better and more energetic?
Celebrating even a few inches that have already melted off?
Posting a picture of what you want to look like in 6 months?
Perhaps it is reading inspirational quotes.
Find whatever it is, and use these things to motivate yourself on a daily basis.
For some folks, watching a TV show like "The Biggest Loser" will be majorly motivational.
Healthy cooking shows that give you ideas for healthier food choices is another good idea.
Reading and implementing healthy but tasty new recipes helps keep me on track.

Inject some humor!

Laughing is not only a great stress reliever; it also burns calories! Find ways to laugh every day - even if it is laughing at yourself (in a positive way of speaking, of course)! I read a saying on a wall hanging that always gives me a chuckle. It's all about good intentions. it goes something like this:
"I decided to pick up jogging to lose weight but I had to stop because my thighs kept rubbing together and caught my pantyhose on fire!"

Quotes, jokes, ideas and simply everyday chuckles are

important during your journey to weight loss and renewed health. Don't take yourself too seriously - lighten up and laugh a little! And remember: You are more powerful than that cookie calling to you from the kitchen!!!

Deal Enhancers

*Y*ou probably know some things that help you stick with a new plan or goal you have set for yourself. But it never hurts to review a list of deal enhancers!

The following are some of the most powerful deal enhancers you can implement. Decide how many you want to put into place, and then go for it!

- Have a friend join you
- Accountability - keep someone aware of your progress at regular, specified intervals
- Written goals and benchmarks
- Before and after pictures and/or videos
- Journal the process and your progress

The list is short – but oh, so powerful! Choosing even 2 or 3 of these deal enhancers can make all the difference in your healthy living plan! But as we know, things don't always go according to plan. So let's talk in the next chapter about Dealing with Detours. One of my favorite stories is coming right up!

Dealing With Detours...

J've been taking care of my teenage daughter this week - she is recovering from oral surgery. She can only eat things like pudding, mashed potatoes, milkshakes and ice cream. In her boredom, she looks up recipes online for all kinds of carb loaded goodies, and then sends me to the grocery store to get the ingredients to whip together these pound producing preparations!

I've decided something - if I say no to everything, she gets discouraged. So at least I'll try to eat relatively healthy carbs (when I have them) during the occasional "cheat" day. Today was one such day. She found a recipe for "crash hot potatoes" from a lady who calls herself the "Pioneer Woman". The recipe was easy enough, albeit a bit time intensive.

We ran out of olive oil long before dear daughter felt we had enough to adorn those special spuds in all of their glory. So she used butter. Lots of it. She also loaded them (and I DO mean loaded) with salt - Celtic Sea Salt, to be exact (a coarse, mineral-loaded salt from the sea). Fresh ground pepper was added to top off the look.

My first sniff of trouble came when I smelled something funny coming from the oven. I opened it up to find streams of rich creamy butter pouring off the sides of the cookie sheet (I had no idea how much she used). I dabbed what I could with a damp cloth (off the oven door) and put them back in.

A few minutes later, when I went to take them out, I noticed a small problem. The dripping butter had created a flaming fire in the bottom of the oven!

"What are you going to do now??" dear daughter asked nervously.

I took out the potatoes with an oven mitt, grabbed the baking soda, and shook it onto the fire. Presto. Fire out.

But did that smoke spoil those crispy, buttery, salty rich Crash Hot Potatoes? No, indeed!

The first delectable bite was proof enough.

Trouble was, I had difficulty stopping at one small potato. And two. Would you believe, about 3 potatoes later, I finally forced myself to put the remainder away?

They were delicious - heavenly - but there was way too much salt added. This in turn, made me extremely thirsty - and I have been painfully parched for several hours now. Seems I can't get enough liquid to balance out the sodium in my cells!

I guess one good thing about it is that I don't think I can eat again tonight! I'm bloated, salted and stuffed like a turkey!

Now there's a lesson to all of this. (You knew that was coming, didn't you?)

Day 3 of my diet, and I "blew it". Right?

WRONG.

I will consider this a "cheat day" as far as low carb count goes.

But it's not a lost cause!

The potatoes were excellent - and although starchy and rather high in carbs, they still are a relatively "natural" food (minus the mega-butter, I suppose!)

I'm aware of how I felt "post-feast" - and taking notes so

I remember this before eating "too much of a good thing" the next time.

Also, I will jump right back on the wagon, and not let this deter me. After all, I'm going to adapt to be somewhat in a celebratory state of mind while she is recovering from painful wisdom tooth extraction. Then after she gets busy again at work and school, my low - carb eating plan will become just a way of life on most days.

What's the lesson in this for you? Don't give up when the detours come! Just because you get off the beaten path (familiar highway) doesn't mean you have to throw the whole thing out the window! Keep cruising and you will reach your destination in time.

Learn from it - enjoy those occasional cheat days or meals, and keep on trucking towards your weight loss goals. You can do it. I believe in you!

Let's take a look next at what may well become your favorite days in every week – your glorious carb cheat days!

CARB CHEAT DAYS -
Planning and Pleasure

*W*hat? I'm talking about carb cheat days right after talking about going low carb?

Well, I must admit that I returned to add this section after I nearly completed the book so that I could tell you what happened with me, as well as some popular thought roaming around the diet and fitness world right now. There are 2 really tough things about going low carb every day as a lifestyle.

1) It's hard to maintain!

2) The body adjusts and adapts to its current eating habits and may restrict weight loss after a time because it acts as a kind of "set point" unless you change something up.

So, you may have heard about taking carb cheat days to keep the body "confused", if you will. But before you rush off to gorge on cake, pasta and ice cream, please pay close attention!

First, you'll need to find what works best for your body. I suggest starting with one of these two options, but follow the plan, and also keep tracking to see how your body responds.

Option 1: Take a carb cheat day every 3-4 days

Option 2: Take a carb cheat day every 7 days

But here's the dynamic deal associated with whichever option you choose: **Eat healthy carbs!**

One of the ways I often feel deprived on a traditional "low carb diet" is that I am denied perfectly healthy foods - like sweet potatoes, apples, brown rice, and many other fresh fruits, vegetables and legumes that God created for our pleasure!

So, add in your carb cheat days. Try both options 1 and

2 above, and track your results. But on those carb cheat days, load up on healthy carbs and feel good about doing it!

Stay away from sugar, white flour products and white rice. Stick with your wide, colorful array of fresh fruits and vegetables, beans and legumes, whole grains and healthy sweeteners. And really enjoy yourself with those comfort foods on your special days!

I had to add in this section, because after some such "carb cheat days" that I allowed myself to take, I actually LOST weight the following day! So try it out with joy, and see with what frequency your body responds most favorably. I can assure you that this plan will be *exponentially easier to stick with* than simply gritting your teeth and trying to maintain low carb every single day of your life.

Good Carbs = Good Feelings = Good Results!

Another thing you will want to understand is how to figure out "net carbs". You may have noticed the term "net carbs" on various packaged food at the store. It's really simple. Net carbs are total carbs per serving minus the fiber content. So when I eat a slice of Ezekiel bread, for instance, it has 15 carbs per slice, but 3 grams of fiber. Thus, my net carbs for that slice of whole grain bread is just 12 g. (15-3).

Fiber is a very good thing as it even helps lower your carb load! More on fiber is coming in the Fabulous Fiber chapter – just following the next chapter!

DEAL-Tweakers

There are so many variations that you can try once you get on track with losing pounds and inches.

At various times of my life, I've followed different plans - such as Fit For Life (food combining book), predominately raw food (50-75%), the Eat Right For Your Type guidelines, and others, I'm sure.

I've found some of it helpful, other suggestions have not been so practical for me. You've likely encountered a similar experience if you have dieted for any length of time.

Find what works with your body - as you gain more "body awareness", especially by tracking in your food journal how your body responds to various foods, you will come up with a good system well suited for you.

I personally have had big results from adding more raw foods to my diet, with resulting high energy and mental clarity. I've also noted huge results when I removed wheat from my daily diet - which resulted in the disappearance of tummy bloat!

Raw Foods

Rah,Rah,Raw!

Since I have had such marvelous results whenever I increase my percentage of raw foods, I have to mention this. I'm sure there is a book coming on this topic alone!

When my oldest son, Jesse, was just a little tyke, I was stressing to him the importance of eating raw foods. I said to him one day while standing in front of the refrigerator:

"Jesse, did you know that raw foods are really good for you?"

"Raw?" he questioned in his little boy voice.

"Yes, raw." I replied. They are very, very good for helping you grow up to be big and strong."

With a puzzled glance, he looked up at me again, with his fist pumping in the air and questioned: "You mean like, rah, rah, rah?"

I laughed - realizing he confused RAW with a cheering term.

But when you think about it, RAW food does cause the body to cheer!

Here's why:

Benefits of Raw Foods

Raw foods have live enzymes that all of your body processes need to function optimally

Raw food is packed with nutrition

Raw food is more filling than processed junk foods

Raw foods are more satisfying

Raw foods are great for your skin

…And the list goes on!

You'll start craving them once you get cleaned out and start feeding REAL Food to your body!

(I'm craving fresh apple juice something fierce about now)

Shoot to increase the amount of raw foods in your diet.

You can start small, but give yourself a challenge as well. What about going for 25% raw in your diet this week?

If you generally eat 4 smaller meals a day, that's just one raw meal, or 25% of each meal can be raw foods.

Calculating % of Raw Foods In Your Diet

Here's an easy way to measure this.

Let's say I have a big salad plus a piece of roasted chicken for lunch today.

My meal was half chicken, half salad - so I ate 50% raw.

* Beside each meal that you are tracking, you can write down the % of raw food you ate at that meal.

Add the % of raw foods consumed that day and divide by the number of meals you ate for the total.

Here's an example:

Today, let's say you ate 4 meals.

Breakfast - (shake) - 33% raw (1/3 of your ingredients were raw fruit, for instance)

Lunch - Large salad with raw sunflower seeds - 100% raw

Snack - Organic Banana with natural roasted almond butter - 50% raw

Supper - Chicken, rice, steamed broccoli and slaw - 25% raw

Here's how you will calculate the result:

You ate 4 meals.

Now add up the raw amount you ate: 33% + 100% + 50% + 25% = 208%

208 divided by 4 (meals) = 52% raw for the day.

See how easy that was?

If you begin increasing your amount of raw foods daily, you will be amazed at how you will begin not only to LOOK better, but to feel more amazing as well!

Fabulous Fiber

Fiber is Crucial to Good Health

Are you getting what you need?

Fiber is crucial to our diet because;

- it helps regulate the digestive system by adding bulk that keeps you "regular"

- It helps you feel fuller, thus cutting down on the amount of calories you eat

- Naturally found in fruits and vegetables, this is one of the first places you suffer when eating primarily processed and packaged foods

The Recommended Daily Allowance (RDA) for fiber is 25 -38g daily.

Most of us are WOEFULLY lacking in fiber because of the multitudinous portions of processed foods we consume on a daily basis on what we call the Standard American Diet -SAD). And it is SAD!

In fact, Wikipedia says that the average American gets 50% or less of the recommended allowance of fiber each day, and that when considering the fast food junk consumed by the average teenager in the USA, it may be as low as 20%! This in turn can lead to obesity and many other health issues. So, what's the fiber content in a typical day of food?

Breakfast - Egg McMuffin or bacon and eggs with white

toast / coffee - 2 g

Lunch:

Burger and fries (you're in a rush) - 8g (if you're fortunate)

Snack: a candy bar (or masked candy bar, such as most granola bars or "protein" bars) - you're dragging around 3 pm and just need something to get you to supper!

Supper: Fried Chicken

Mashed potatoes and gravy - 3g

Corn on the side - 2g

Biscuits or rolls

Slaw or a small salad (you're proud of yourself for eating raw!) - 2g

Dessert: a piece of pie or cake - 1g

Late night munchies:

Of course, your body didn't get much real nutrition with the typical food fare you fed it today, so now you're hungry again. You decide to reward yourself for a hard day's work by sitting down with a bowl (or two) or ice cream while watching one of your favorite TV shows. (0-1g fiber)

Does the above scenario sound all too familiar?

The average amount of fiber in the food fare above is___ (on a good day, about 18g.) That is much less than even the RDA (which may be on the very minimum side, anyway!) It's quite possible that your consumption of SAD (Standard American Diet) is giving you up to twice as many calories as you need, half (or less) of the fiber you require for maximum functioning, AND (believe it or not) scant nutrition.

Now you know why (crazy as it sounds) you might feel hungry a couple of hours after eating fast food - or even a heavy dinner meal.... your body is still crying out for the nutrients it needs to function properly! Why not give it what it is craving - REAL foods - with an increasing amount of raw foods - particularly fruits and vegetables (organic, if possible). You can "kill two birds with one stone", as they say. Eat healthy foods that give you both nutrients AND fiber!

<u>Sample Fiber-Full and Healthy Meal Plan for the day</u>

Let's take a look at a day of healthier fare - and see how it measures up in the fiber department.

Breakfast: A bowl of whole grain oats with 1 c fresh raspberries (12 g. fiber)

Snack: A handful of sunflower seeds and raisins (about 5 g. fiber)

Lunch: A Large Salad with fresh peppers, cucumbers, carrots and romaine lettuce (about 5 g. or so fiber)

1 slice Ezekiel (sprouted grain) bread with natural peanut butter (about 4 g. fiber)

Afternoon snack: 1 c. blueberries and strawberries (about 3 g. fiber)

Dinner:

Grilled Chicken

Asian Slaw (1 c - about 3 g. fiber)

Steamed Broccoli (3/4 c fresh - 7 g. of fiber)

That is approximately 39 g. of fiber for the day! It's amazing to see how a few simple changes can create massive effects in the health and fiber departments!

UPDATE: Ok, folks - it's been a month now. I've followed the DEAL with some mishaps - including a business trip out of state where I was so busy, I didn't take the time to write down what all I was eating! (In retrospect, that's probably a good thing).

I also had visions (you have too, I venture) of swimming in the hotel swimming pool to get that much needed exercise while I was gone. Well… you can imagine that by the time our sessions ended and we had eaten, I was so exhausted I didn't make the effort to go swimming! Still, I must 'fess up to my results. Remember, I didn't do so well on the trip - and I've taken some "carb cheat" days, and we've had some birthdays and celebrations (I'm the queen of 'legitimate' excuses).Still, I've lost a total of 5 pounds in the past month. (I gained about 3 on that trip I mentioned!) I didn't lose 10, but 5 pounds are gone.

Now you might be thinking - "That's not so great! What's she bragging about?" And that's EXACTLY what I would be thinking too - had I not measured my body to begin with, and continued to track each area for small to moderate changes. I'm telling you why this is VITALLY important! I lost another 5 1/2" in the past two weeks! That brings my one month total to: *Lost:* 5 pounds. (80 oz!) *Lost:* 14 1/2"

And I still have consistent exercise to add to this picture! Do you think I can continue to be motivated after seeing those inches (that aren't) in black and white? You betcha I am! And the same will be true for you. Pounds alone are not a reliable measure of how your body is changing and readapting over time. So track those inches - and watch them disappear.

Celebrate your victories, and no matter how much you might blow it on any given day, get up the next day and get rolling again! Do the DEAL, track not only your intake, but track your measurements every couple of weeks, and reward yourself with something you love to do. If I can do this, YOU CAN, TOO!

Another Great DEAL for Tracking Fat Loss and BMI

I'm sure you've heard of it - body mass index is a way of measuring the percentage of your body that is currently fat. They have scales that supposedly measure this (I have a pair - they're not reliable). In addition, you may have heard or read of using "body calipers" or fat calipers, to pinch the inches of fat on various parts of your body. While supposedly more accurate, you really need someone else's help to reach your back areas - and that can be downright EMBARRASSING!

Apart from this, our alternative perhaps has been to go to the local gym and have a trainer use their fancy equipment to track our current BMI.

Well, I'm thrilled to say I've discovered a simple alternative that is said to be quite accurate - and it will help you track both your % of body fat and your current body mass index (BMI)! It's called a Fat Loss Monitor (the particular brand I own is Omron), and it is a simple handheld device. It comes with instructions as well as a handy-dandy laminated sheet that gives the guidelines for low, normal, high and very high readings for your age and sex - both for % of fat and for BMI.

I've found this extremely helpful for consistent tracking of my fat loss. In addition, I'm able to see before my eyes that "healthy" fat doesn't make you fatter! My daily diet typically includes flax oil, organic coconut oil, and olive oil, but the fat loss monitor is showing steady improvement - lowering - of the all-important numbers!

I encourage you to purchase one of these for your "weight loss toolkit" when you can - the one I purchased cost about $45. Well worth it, in my humble opinion!

Food Substitutions for the Stuff You Crave

Chocolate!

Ok - so Hershey bars are a thing of the past. How on earth will you live without chocolate? Believe it or not, you don't have to! Now I know, that some in the health arena will tell you to cut out all chocolate - it's simply not good for you (they say). And it does have theobromine in it - which is a stimulant that gives you energy similar to your coffee kick in the morning. Chocolate does have some caffeine - so try some and gauge your body's reaction to it. If you have bursts of energy with no harmful side effects, then why not have your chocolate fix and enjoy it! Just leave out the processed sugar and flour, and you'll be all the healthier for it!

And I say again, why not have chocolate if your body doesn't react negatively to it? Just go for the GOOD stuff! I bought a glorious bag of Organic Cacao - packed with vitamins and antioxidants - and wow, is it heavenly to sniff!

But do I only sniff it? Nope. I use that stuff and enjoy every second of it! It is not processed with Alkali (like the cocoa you buy at the grocery store), and it is rich, delicious and good for you! If you can't locate any in your hometown, you can find some through the Amazon marketplace. The kind I purchased is raw, organic, and filled with antioxidants, iron and magnesium. In addition, it has many health benefits, including flavanols, polyphenols, 100% cacao, and is cold pressed! AND - did you know that raw cacao powered is also a good source of fiber?

I don't know about you, but I just discovered a bullet list of reasons why I CAN enjoy my chocolate without guilt! And now, you can too!

Here's my all time favorite way to use my organic cacao in the morning:

Chocolate Protein Shake for Breakfast

Ingredients:

3-5 ice cubes

1 cup purified water /

4-8 oz unsweetened almond milk

1/2 frozen banana chunks (optional)

1 1/2 scoops vegetable protein

1 tsp all natural peanut butter (unsweetened)

1 heaping tsp Cacao powder

1 packet of Stevia powdered sweetener

1 Tb flax oil (optional)

2 tsp ground flaxseed

1/2 tsp pure vanilla extract (optional)

*P*ut all ingredients into a Magic Bullet Cup (or blender, if you don't own a Magic Bullet). Mix until well blended. Taste for adequate sweetness. Consume and enjoy!

Now, some of you are wondering why on earth I add some of the ingredients listed above. So, to calm your inquiring minds, I'd like to tell you! The ice and/or frozen bananas make the consistency like a icee or milkshake. Yum!

The almond milk is optional - sometimes I use just water. But almonds are high in protein, low in carbs, and add a silky texture to the shake.The protein powder helps keep me fuller longer, and also adds healthy amino acids to my system to start my day right. I use my all time favorite pea protein powder for this purpose.The peanut butter (Kroger brand has ranked high for taste, so I use that) is low in carbs, but adds a yummy taste and creaminess to it. The Cacao powder gives your shake that chocolaty yummy-ness - and gives you not only a kick in the morning, but adds antioxidants as well!

The Flax Oil (Spectrum Naturals is one brand) is a healthy oil that actually helps you lose weight, as opposed to so many of the processed oils that make you gain weight - keep it refrigerated and use it up within about a month. It's buttery flavor blends in beautifully with the shake - you won't even taste the oil in it! (If you prefer, simply skip the oil and use flaxseeds instead)

* *Hint:* In the winter months especially, you may want to pick up the flax oil with added natural Vitamin D - and enjoy that one-two punch of healthiness in one bottle.

The fresh ground flaxseed (I grind organic whole flaxseeds in the Magic Bullet ahead of time and keep them in the refrigerator) adds fiber to your shake, as well as giving you even more flax benefits from this small powerhouse of a seed.

Stevia is a natural plant used for sweetening and is native to South America (although you may be able to find a plant to put in your garden for summer growing). It is low in carbs, but quite sweet, and you can use it without fear of artificial chemicals and negative body and brain reactions (aspartame is a nightmare for the brain according to some researchers!) - and it is so simple to pour a packet into your shake. Look in the health food section for a brand that is not heavily processed and doesn't add additional sucrose or dextrose sweeteners.

So, there you have it. This is my morning routine. I simply vary between chocolate/peanut butter shakes, and occasionally will have a fruit based shake. This morning, I used ice cubes and frozen peaches instead of the cacao powder and peanut butter. What a simple, fast and delicious way to start the day! It might seem like a lot of ingredients - and you can trim it down as you wish. Experiment! Find your own variations! But I can tell you - once I have my flaxseeds ground and waiting for me in the fridge, it probably takes me under 3 minutes to put the ingredients together and whip up my breakfast. I absolutely LOVE it!

Shortcut hint: - Toss whole flaxseeds into your shake and let the blender grind them for you while you blend your shake.

Healthy DEAL Recipes

Quick and Easy Power Packed Cole Slaw

1-2 bags of organic broccoli slaw (or cabbage)

1 c. organic purple cabbage, shredded or cut into thin strips (optional)

1 tsp celery seed

1/4 c. Asian Salad Dressing (I tried Annie's Organic Asian Sesame)

1/4 tsp Stevia (if you like it a little sweeter) - or Agave Syrup

1/4 c. raw slivered almonds or sunflower seeds (optional) - or fresh sesame seeds!

This is a breeze to whip up if you purchase a healthy salad dressing in a bottle.

Simply put all the ingredients in a bowl. Shake the dressing and then add to taste. Mix this up and put it in the refrigerator for a couple of hours or so, to meld the flavors. Delicious!!

Salmon Patties

1 can pink salmon
1/2 c. ground oats (or oatmeal)
2 Tb lemon juice (or lemon pepper spice)
1 egg (optional) - or use 1/3 c. ground flaxseed to bind seasonings

Pour out the salmon and juice into a bowl. Smash with a fork, being sure to also crush the soft bones (full of calcium!). Add the ground oatmeal, the lemon juice or lemon pepper, and the egg or flaxseed.

Season to taste. Seasonings may include southwest chipotle, Italian herbs or dressing, or simply salt and pepper to taste. Grill or fry in pan in Coconut oil to taste. Flip over after the first side is browned. Yum!

Dealing with Seasons of Sacrifice

*H*ave you ever given anything up "for Lent"? I remember hearing about other kids in elementary school do this, and it was foreign to me. The church I attended did not observe Lent, so it seemed rather strange. But I think it has plenty of merit now that I'm older!

Lent is the period of time leading up to the death and subsequent resurrection of Jesus Christ. It was looked upon as a time of sacrifice - giving up something you normally would consume - in order to focus on the sacrifice that Christ made for us on the cross. Common sacrifices of foods included red meat, dairy products, and other various foods.

The observation of Lent was intended to provide time and space for meditation, and was a time of personal reflection in relation to the way one's life was being lived. Traditionally, the Lenten fast was broken on or just before Easter Sunday, which marks Christ's resurrection from the dead. So what does Lent have to do with you?

If you choose, you can observe Lent as well. It could be during the typical season (from Ash Wednesday to just before Easter Sunday), or you might choose another time. It has been said that a "fast" from food (or anything else that can be addictive such as technology, for instance) will show you in a hurry how dependent you actually are upon these things!

I decided to seriously observe Lent this year. I've been feeling for some time that there were certain foods that I should give up for a time, to see how my body responds. While many people choose one item, I decided to cut out three different things from my diet during this approximately 45-day period. What did I decide to give up?
I chose meat, wheat and sugar.

I know - it seems extreme, as some of my friends have told me. And although I'm not bragging about it (which defeats the purpose), I find it simple to tell a friend if we're eating out or something, that I cannot eat these things because I've given them up for Lent. Amazingly, I don't get the type of pressure I feel when I just tell someone I'm giving it up because I'm "going on a diet"!

In addition to the above, while I am not specifically denying myself dairy products and eggs, I am trying to avoid them as much as possible. Dairy products tend to make my nose stuffy, and sometimes they make my stomach feel heavy. Gauge your own reactions to various foods and begin to track how you feel after you eat certain things. Your "Lenten List" may look different from mine.

So how hard is it? I've eaten out once since I began, and it wasn't too difficult! The only thing that "may" have had an offending ingredient was the salad dressing at the restaurant, but since I don't know for sure and I wasn't going to ask for the ingredient listing, I just chose a "go with the flow" attitude.

Surprisingly, actually making the decision to finally take the jump - and then explaining my reasons if someone asks, has freed me up to keep the fast. Do I see results yet? Yes, I do!

I've suspected for a long time that wheat was creating problems with me, but it is so prevalent in so many foods that it's hard to get away from it.

Wheat (gluten allergy) is a BIG problem, and wheat can cause inflammation in body systems - leading to all kinds of disorders in the system. Most of the wheat consumed in these days is a hybrid of the original grain. Today's modern wheat has been coined more of a "weed" than a true grain. Sugar, of course, is an ever-insidious enemy, stealing the health and vibrancy of so many. It is processed so extensively from its original form, that the body sees it more as a chemical than a food. I have a nephew who determined to give up sugar - the only change he made to his diet - and lost over 50 pounds!!

What about the meat? I know from study about digestion that meat takes the body a LONG time to digest - in some cases up to 3 days. I also know that we can get proper nutrients without eating meat, and that much of our meat supply is loaded with hormones and antibiotics. In fact, because of a severe reaction, I have not been able to eat beef for some 15 years.

I'm used to eating a lot of chicken, but I'm giving that up for now. I do have fish, so the grilled catfish I enjoyed the other night when I ate out with a friend, as well as the salmon patties

I make at home, are a nice diversion. I could sense changes in my body pretty quickly. Within 3 days, I lost about 3 pounds. I'm not kidding!

There are still plenty of foods I can have, I just need to get creative and try some different things. This has given me more time for focused meditation on God, on the direction my life is supposed to take, as well as time to explore some different recipes without the above ingredients. And I'm enjoying it! I can feel the structure of my body changing - particularly around my stomach and hips. After 45 days, I may not want to go back! I will also admit, that since I cut out these items, I'm not paying super close attention to my carb consumption - as long as it is a "natural" product, it qualifies for feeding purposes.

I've also noticed that my "full meter" seems to be reset. I'm not famished like I felt like I was before - I believe this is because my body is finally getting natural nutrients and isn't screaming for "more, more, more" since the items I used to eat were lacking so much in nutritional value.

For example, did you know that processed (white) sugar, wheat (pasta, flour, etc.), and rice actually STEAL B vitamins out of your body in order to digest them? Since B vitamins are the energy vitamins, no wonder we get so tired when we eat a meal heavy in any of these substances! I'm also using this time to study, learn and experiment more with raw foods - with full plans to release a (raw) cookbook in the near future sharing what I've learned! (If you don't cook it, what do we call it - a Rawbook?)

I've already discovered an absolutely delicious recipe for flourless crackers - which, when doused with natural peanut butter, promptly satisfy my cravings for crackers with crunch, with a hint of salt and mega healthy nutrition!

I've heard and read about so many people who dropped stubborn weight effortlessly once they began to eat raw - even 50% raw can make a big difference! So, watch for more to come on that in the near future.

What about a raw organic chocolate bar recipe? Can be used in milkshakes, for chocolate chips, or by the bite! YUM!!! (Just don't overdo it - this is a powerful antioxidant feel good snack!)

I sense you would be terribly disappointed if I didn't include the recipe I have tweaked for this heavenly homemade chocolate bar. Take a peek near the end of the book for the riveting recipe!

Dairy Diversions

Dairy Reactions are Not Uncommon

Yesterday, I had my son and his friend and wife over for Sunday dinner. We decided to go Mexican. So we had burritos with roasted chicken, refried beans, black beans and cheese. I had fresh guacamole and sweet peppers on the table to add, as well as our favorite, Pace Medium Picante Salsa.

In addition, we had tortilla chips with cheese dip, which I heated in a small crock-pot. It was a hit!!

Although I have been avoiding dairy, I decided to indulge yesterday. I noticed it as early as last night. I was coughing before I went to bed (dairy products are mucus producing), and I felt rather bloated. This morning, the scales told the rest of the story! Up a pound or so, and feeling bloated. So today, I decided to get back to dairy free and low carb.

I began with my typical protein shake for breakfast - this time with fresh almond milk. (I made it last evening). The taste was a bit different from store bought almond milk, but it was good and filling. I noticed more energy for my work in the morning hours today! Since I'm so busy in the office today, I decided on a quick lunch. An egg sandwich sounded good! So I looked to see what I could "throw together" for a tasty, but quick sandwich. What I came up with was even better than I hoped for!

Easy Dairy Free Recipe

I found a couple of mini bags of chopped peppers (from last season) in my freezer. One bag was HOT (which I discovered after the first bite). Good! I had a nice surprise!

I put a tsp or so of sesame oil in the skillet and added the peppers. I warmed those and sautéed them briefly and then whipped up 3 eggs in a bowl with a fork. I added that mixture to the skillet and then sprinkled it with Celtic Sea Salt and smoked paprika (yum!) I flipped the mixture when it was cooked on the bottom, and then gave it a few more minutes until it was cooked through. And what did I use for the sandwich part? I simply washed two organic romaine leaves, patted them dry, and sliced the egg round lengthwise to fit on the leaf. I added a squeezed strip of organic mayonnaise, and freshly ground pepper. Then I added a covering of fresh sliced cucumber. I covered that with the other lettuce leaf, breathed a prayer of thanks, and crunched away! My, but it was delicious! The hot peppers added such a punch, that I did not miss any cheese in the least! (And yes, I still have grated cheese sitting in my fridge from yesterday)

You can play around with all kinds of additions and spices/ or herbs, but here's what I tried today and absolutely loved:

1 tsp (or so) sesame oil

2-3 TB chopped peppers (fresh or frozen)

3 eggs, beaten

Sea Salt

Black Pepper

Smoked Paprika

For the sandwich:

Fresh organic romaine leaves, washed (or substitute your choice of seaweed sheets)

Toppings:

Organic mayonnaise (optional mustard)
Fresh sliced cucumbers

See the paragraphs just above for cooking and preparation directions.

I had two "sandwiches", and they were absolutely delicious! I still have half of my eggs left for another sandwich tomorrow. I feel full, happy and lean for my next few hours of work, too. That was one amazing low carb but high taste entree!

We've talked a lot about the yummy stuff that is going IN you, but what about what is ON you? Turn the page and find out the surprising truth!

Here's the DEAL With Clothing

So, you may already have started the DEAL and are noticing positive changes. What about your wardrobe?

If you're like many of us, you didn't give away all of those smaller sizes of clothing - telling yourself that you'd get back into them one day soon! Whether you did - or didn't - get rid of all but your current clothing size, here's something to keep in mind. Let me explain by way of a true story (mine)! Last Wednesday, I was getting dressed for a business meeting, and decided I would wear a pair of gray dress slacks with a blue sweater. It looked professional enough on the hangers! But when I put on the slacks…. they just didn't look right. Yes, they were a little baggy in the seat, but the waist fit ok. Why didn't they look right?

I finally took them off and picked up a pair of black pants that were a smaller size. I quickly tried them on and looked in the mirror. I was AMAZED at what I saw! I kid you not - I looked like I had instantly lost about 10 pounds!

That is the difference you will see as well between slightly baggy clothing and nicely fitted clothes. Keep those smaller sized clothing articles at hand and try them on often. If you gave them all away, then just go shopping for a short while and try on some smaller sizes there to see what you think. Not only will you look a lot trimmer in items that are fitted to your new body, but it will also give you more inspiration to keep on keeping on with your new eating plan!

I'm enjoying many of those items I "grew out of" over the past couple of years - because now they are fitting again!

Oh, and on an inspirational note: If any of you are procrastinating the cleaning of your closet because of all the decision making it will require, simply have your teenaged daughter on hand to critique your clothing options. I promise it will be motivating to get rid of those out of style items once she has her say! (And, if you don't happen to have a teenaged daughter, simply hire one to help you make decisions for a few hours - you'll have a lot to donate - trust me!)

More Amazing Recipes

Tuna Salad "Sandwich"

I really enjoy tuna from time to time. But what do you do about the taste without the sweet relish? (Traditional relish is packed with sugar and artificial dyes).

I've found a solution.

Here is my simple (but delicious) recipe:

1-2 packets of water packed tuna (no extra juice)

1-2 TB organic mayonnaise

1/4 tsp celery seed (or 1/4 c. chopped OG celery)

1/4 tsp dill weed (amazing relish taste!)

Optional ingredients:

Shredded OG carrots

Chopped OG boiled eggs

Fresh or frozen green peas

Mix ingredients together with a fork and adjust seasonings to taste. Spoon onto Organic Romaine lettuce leaves to make a sandwich, or wrap in seaweed wrappers. Also, making a tuna salad on baby spinach leaves is a very tasty treat!

Super Quick Energy Snack

Organic Banana

1 Tsp natural peanut butter (no sugar) or almond butter.

Peel ripened banana. Spread with natural peanut butter or almond butter and consume.

Delicious! (Sometimes I have this for my lunch or a mid afternoon snack)

Organic Homemade Chocolate Bar Bliss

*T*his is my own version - adapted from a recipe I found online on a chocolate blog called "Chocolate Covered Katie" - and boy, is it amazing!

1/2 cup + 1 TB organic cacao powder

3 TB melted organic coconut oil (warmed in the oven or dehydrator or steamed in a bowl over a pan of hot water)

1/4 cup organic erythritol, or less stevia to taste

1 tsp pure vanilla extract

1/8-1/4 c. almond or coconut milk (for a lighter "milk chocolate") - optional

Whisk ingredients together in a small bowl until very smooth. Spread in a flat rectangular container and freeze. Break into chunks by "cutting" with a table knife. Homemade raw chocolate - does it get any better than this?

Note: This can also be broken and used as chocolate chips in various recipes.

Super Easy Leftover Bean Soup

*D*o you hate throwing out small portions of leftovers? Me, too. I decided to try something different. Whenever I had some leftover beans and corn, I froze the remainder to make some warm soup for a cool day. We had one such spring day, and I pulled out my crock-pot and opened the freezer.

Anything bean or corn-like qualified to be tossed into the mix!

I added:

Leftover beans

Corn "broth"

Leftover corn

1 can of organic "Tri - Bean Blend"

1 TB of dried organic vegetable flakes (from the health food store)

1 tsp. Blackened Blend seasoning (also from the health food store)

1 or 2 bay leaves (optional)

I simply dropped in both the frozen and fresh items, added the herbs, stirred, and put the Crockpot on high to cook. I smelled it soon enough!

It was the most heavenly bean soup I have ever tasted in my life! It was seriously AH-mazing!

I had 3 bowls the first evening.

Don't be afraid to try new things, even leftovers in your freezer from those "not quite finished" meals. You just may be amazed at the result!

SweetHeat Veggie Asian Stir Fry

1-2 garlic cloves, minced

2-3 TB sesame oil

Optional hot chili oil

1-2 cups chopped zucchini

1-2 bags broccoli or traditional slaw

½ cup organic carrot sticks

1 c. broccoli (optional)

8 mushrooms, washed and sliced

Any variety of other vegetables, optional

* 1-2 c. bean threads or sweet potato noodles

*H*eat oil in skillet or large pan. Add garlic and mushrooms, and then add the longer- cooking veggies such as carrots and broccoli. Add the remaining veggies and stir while frying.

Mix the following sauce with a whisk and add to the skillet:

1/3 c. Bragg's Liquid Aminos (or soy sauce)

Fresh grated ginger or 1 tsp powdered ginger

1-2 Tb pure maple syrup or agave syrup

Add sauce to the skillet once the veggies are mostly cooked. Add the noodles (bean threads or sweet potato noodles if you're avoiding wheat) and stir together. Taste and continue to season as needed to get a tasty balance of sweet, heat and salt.

Serve on a plate or in a bowl with a fork or chopsticks. This makes amazing leftovers as well!

* Sweet Potato noodles can be found at Oriental or Korean grocery stores

Tropical Dream Supreme Juice

2 pears

1 large mango

1/4 fresh pineapple

Peel fruit unless it is organic. Remove brown outer skin from pineapple.

Run through a juicer. Enjoy!

I made the leftover juice into ice pops by pouring into freezer molds.

Since the leftover pulp was rather creamy, I decided to spread it out on a Paraflexx sheet and dehydrate it in my Excalibur dehydrator. After drying for several hours on about 110 degrees, I flipped the sheet over and peeled off the leather onto a regular dehydrating sheet. Then I dried it for another hour or so until the "fruit leather" was to desired consistency. Yum!

The DEAL Recapped

So you've read the book and learned all about the DEAL way of living. It's easy to remember, and really pretty easy to follow, particularly if you focus on adding many more raw natural foods to your diet, and you keep your carb cheat days in their place!

Now it's time to kick it into gear! Don't let this be just another "good idea" that collects dust on the cyber library shelf of your mind. Actually put it into action! Become aware of what your body responds favorably to, and what makes you feel bloated and lethargic.

Follow the DEAL and tweak it to fit your particular needs and goals, and then watch the magic happen!

Remember the Acrostic?

D - Detox

E - Exercise

A - Action Tracking

L - Low Carb

I challenge you to give this at least 60 days of focus, track and measure your results and then go from there. You can be on your way to a brand new you!

I've enjoyed this so much, and as I continue to experiment with recipes and healthy food choices, I promise I will share them with you in upcoming books. Keep your eyes peeled for

The DEAL Cookbook Series, which will be released soon, and will be fun and helpful companion volumes to this book.

Until then my friend, DEAL your way into a brand new future full of health and promise!

— **Megan C. Scott**

Meet the Author

Megan C. Scott is a writer, author, speaker and coach. She enjoys cooking, creating, and (of course) eating! She is a mom to 4 and Grandma to 2, and loves to spend time with family and friends. Her goal it to help as many people as possible to enjoy both their food and their health - without super restrictive, boring dieting.

She says "no" to starvation or fancy diets, and "yes" to the best taste and goodness that God's bountiful produce provides for us to enjoy.

Megan ate a typical "Standard American Diet" (SAD for short) until she was about 16 years of age. At that time, she encountered various health issues including low blood sugar, or hypoglycemia. She began a quest to research a way to treat her symptoms with food, rather than drugs. All these years later, she still believes that food is the best medicine!

She is ever searching for healthy, easy to prepare foods that will boost both health and energy. And she loves to share them with her readers!

Megan would love to keep in touch with you! Visit her (and contact her) on her website: https://HealthyWeightLossAndFatBurning.com and be sure to sign up for your free gift while you are there.

Thank you for your interest in the Here's the DEAL series,

and be sure to keep a copy of the flagship book close at hand to maintain your motivation!

Remember to watch for upcoming volumes of recipes that will inspire you to stick to the DEAL and reach your weight loss goals in less time than you may have dreamed. Life is good!

Conclusion

There you have it. The simple DEAL blueprint plan that can help you reach your weight loss and fat burning goals without boring, bland diet foods!

Only the tastiest recipes make the cut into the Here's the DEAL books.

I would love to hear from you!

Be sure to **snag your free DEAL recipes PDF book** and sign up to my email list to get **healthy living tips, recipes, upcoming book release notifications and more!**

Simply follow the link below to sign up for your bonus gift:
https://healthyweightlossandfatburning.com/BonusRecipesGift

And please take just a moment to turn the page and leave a review for this book. I appreciate it so much!

Can you help?

If you enjoyed this recipe book, would you PRETTY PLEASE (with a cherry on top) **leave a review on Amazon?**

Simply visit:
https://healthyweightlossandfatburning.com/DEAL to leave your review.

Reviews are super important to the success of this book. And **your feedback is valued!** So PLEASE take just 2 minutes to leave an honest review now.

Thanks so much - I truly appreciate it!

Other Books by Megan C. Scott

https://healthyweightlossandfatburning.com/EggCitingRecipes

https://healthyweightlossandfatburning.com/SuperShakes&Smoothies